Conte

Hannah's Nursing Journe

Tom's Nursing Journey

Lucy's Nursing Journey

Chapter 11: Student Nurse Tips

Hannah's nursing journey

Chapter 1: First Placement

Three years after I had completed my nursing training, I had decided to write a book with my fellow colleagues about our time as student nurses' in the NHS. Hannah, Thomas, and Louise all came from different backgrounds and entered nursing to make a positive difference to people's lives. Hannah trained after completing her high school diploma, moving from America to London to complete her training. Whilst Tom entered Nursing after feeling unfulfilled in his career as a journalist, and looked for a change in a career where he could make a difference. Louise trained as a nurse following a rapid change in her personal circumstances, she was made redundant and her husband left her one day to raise her children alone.

We wanted to write this book to share our most memorable experiences on placement. The experiences of a student nurse are a unique training journey that can change your life. As a trainee, you are with patients at their darkest moments and share in other patients' recovery. As a student, you could be holding the hand of a dying patient and provide dignified end of life care, to watching a patient make a full recovery following interventions from a range of healthcare professionals. We all agreed whilst writing the book that the life of a student nurse is like a rollercoaster. At times you will feel happy, tired, or tearful, but that driving force to help others, and to provide caring compassionate care always pulled us through. We hope you enjoy reading our honest accounts of our lives as student nurses and gain an insight into our unique training journey.

On my eighteenth birthday, I received a special card from my Grandmother who had passed away a year previously. My Grandmother had left me her entire fortune and home in Camden in London. My Grandmother was a stunt woman in many classic films, and later worked as a director behind the scenes on television. I had always had a close relationship with my Grandmother and visited her every summer and we would attend theme parks together, go to the theatre, and eat together at expensive restaurants.

When my Grandma passed away, I was entering into a very important part of my life. I was about to make an important decision about my future, and I had decided I wanted to train as a nurse and move to London for three years to complete my training. I packed up my belongings into my rusty brown suitcase, and took one final look at my story Edwardian home. As I traveled in the yellow taxicab I watched as my parents stood waving on the sidewalk, waving with tears in their eyes. My mum stood in her flowery yellow summer dress, crying under her large dark oval shades, and my father stood beside her, cradling her trembling hands as he stood in his grey suit.

I was trembling as I sat in the back of the taxi, I was eighteen years old, so shy and reserved, and had never traveled on my own before and I was about to embark on the biggest journey of my life.

I always had a strong interest in working in the medical field, influenced by my sister who worked as a registered physiotherapist, and my brother Arnold, a junior doctor.

My decision to move to England and embark on a nursing course proved to be a very controversial decision, being the youngest in the family I was told that I wouldn't cope, that I would not survive on my own. In a way, my move to England was a form of rebellion and a way for me to move away from the overprotective structure I was under.

I was so nervous as I sat on the plane. On the journey, I sat next to the most annoying woman in the world Mrs. Oxbridge. Mrs Oxbridge was fifty-six, and wore a large orange dress, orange sandals to match with her wild curly red hair. "Hello young lady, tell me about you? Where are you going, what are your plans?" She asked

"I'm traveling to London to study to become a nurse," I murmured. It was then that Mrs. Oxbridge displayed her unusual eccentric behavior, including clasping onto my hand tightly as the plane took off, she began to show me hundreds of photos she took of her birds in her garden. In a desperate plea to escape, I began to close my eyes and pretended to fall asleep.

I arrived in London at 1 pm and took a taxicab to London. I was so petrified as I made my way to my Grandmother's house, already I was homesick, as the wild rain crashed on the roof of the car. I Instantly missed the California sun. I marveled as I entered inside my Grandmother's two-story Edwardian townhouse. In the dining room was a grand white piano, and on the walls were hundreds of photos of her amazing Hollywood career as a stunt woman. The photos included a picture of her standing next to Steven Spielberg at the Oscars, whilst another photo showed her on the set of titanic. Many of the awards she had won were framed on the wall she achieved in starring in over one hundred films. I marveled as I looked around at my Grandmother's home, now my own home. In her mansion was a luxurious dance hall, a swirl pool, and six Victorian bedrooms upstairs.

I claimed my room in the attic overlooking the grand central park, with the family portrait of me with my Grandmother and parents on a beach in California. I was nervous starting my first day at university as a Nursing student.

I woke up the next day and it was a beautiful Sunday morning in January, I could feel my whole-body trembling as I made my way to the London University. I arrived for the university lecture at 9 am. I looked on in awe at the room filled with a range of people from different backgrounds and ages.

Some of the students had just graduated from school, others were career changes, others were experienced health professionals looking for advancements in their careers.

That day we were allocated to a specific group of twelve students. I became friends with three students. Patience was a thirty-eight-year-old woman, originally from Zimbabwe, who had worked as a carer for twenty years. Simon was twenty-four years old and was struggling to find work following the completion of his media degree Then there was Jenny, a nineteen-year-old girl, who worked as a hairdresser prior to starting the career. Jenny was outspoken, wild in her behavior, and openly rude to people she didn't like.

As a group, we became close friends each day Simon, Jenny, and Patience would go to lunch with me and we would talk about our lives. Jenny would always arrive late for each lecture and was often found painting her nails or reading through OK magazine, whilst after a half an hour into the lecture Patience could be found snoring with her head-tilted back. Simon was always studious and sat at the front of the lecture conscientiously.

Many of our lecturers and seminars focused on the communication aspects of nursing and the history of the profession. Whilst the clinical skills sessions involved us directly practicing nursing skills in the clinical rooms with the mannequins. I remember our final clinical session where we had to practice our skills. We practiced taking manual blood pressures, practiced our CPR compressions, and undertook manual pulse rate. Then it happened. Patience had volunteered to take part in the manual handling demonstration, and she lay on the mock hospital bed with a slide sheet on her. It was then that she screamed as she reached for an item in the bed. It was a skeleton's hand, in shock she rolled out of the bed and fell flat onto the floor. We all laughed in unison.

As students, we were all so different and our different backgrounds and career path brought different qualities to the nursing profession. Patience explained that she lived in a poverty-stricken area in Zimbabwe, and would have to walk seven miles each day to the local well. Patience always dreamed of becoming a nurse and completed classes at night school. Patience came from a humble background and was so positive and emphatic about the sufferings of others.

Simon worked in telecommunications prior to starting the nursing course, and developed both his problem-solving skills and time management skills. Jenny had an eccentric personality, and her vibrant outlook on life helped to boost the morale of the other students.

After three months of studying at the university, I received a notification that I would be starting my placement in the general elderly medical ward in a small community hospital.

I remember the morning of my first placement, I was terrified, I stood in the mirror looking on in awe in my pristine white uniform. I was so nervous at eighteen years of age, unsure about the career path I was entering. I sat at the oval table eating my rice Krispies with my satchel next to me filled with pens, a notebook, and a packed lunch. I was so nervous I dropped the milk in the kitchen causing a river to form.

I made my way to the hospital that morning walking through the crowded London streets. It was a beautiful hot summer morning; I was comforted by the sound of the bluebirds chirping in the sky. I arrived at the hospital at 6:50 am and searched nervously through the hospital for my ward. As I entered the general medical ward, I could feel my whole-body tremble. There were three bays, two male bays, and one female bay. As I walked in, I could see the patients were sleeping in their bed, apart from a few elderly patients who were making their way to the toilet. I watched as the nurses were rushing around completing their notes before they handed over the staff. I could hear the observation machines bleeping, and the snores of the patients in the bed. The cook arrived on the ward and I could smell the foul stench of the eggs and bacon.

I walked nervously into the handover room, there was a young nurse sitting, with red rosy cheeks, and her blond curly hair was wrapped in a bun, her name was Lucy she was to be my mentor. The second nurse was Bleina, a forty-year-old nurse from the Philippines, she had long black hair and wore bright blue-rimmed glasses and had a serious expression on her face. The ward manager Hayley sat with a huge cup of coffee. The two healthcare assistants Trudy and Ann were mother and daughter and looked like they were part of the Brady bunch. I could feel my whole-body trembling as I sat in the handover room. I felt confused as the night nurses delivered the handover of the patients. The patients were admitted with a wide range of illnesses from cancer, to COPD, to complications in their diabetes condition. I felt so happy when Hayley introduced me to the other nurses, I felt accepted as part of the team. Lucy introduced herself to me when she was twenty-four and had been a nurse for over a year. Lucy's hair was wrapped in a messy bun and her lipstick was smothered all over her face.

It was then that Lucy introduced me to the male patients on my bay. The first patient was Clive, a ninety-year-old man who was living with terminal lung cancer. He was fast asleep in his bed. The second Patient was Donald, an eighty-five-year-old man, living with Lewy body dementia and was surrounded by his medals from his time in the police. The third patient was Simon, a forty-one-year-old Headteacher admitted with complications in his diabetes condition. The fourth patient was Richard admitted after being found wandering on the street, he had long curly grey hair and did wash for over a year. The fifth patient was Mark an eighty-year-old man admitted following a suicide attempt.

I followed Lucy around the bay like a lap dog, as she completed the drug round asking her hundreds of questions about the patients. It was then that she suggested that I support Clive to the shower for his wash. I nervously walked up to Clive, trembling, as I assisted him out of the bed and walked to the shower room. "Wow not every day that you meet an American!" he beamed. "Tell me about you, what was your career?" I asked.
"I worked as a paramedic for over forty years, when I retired, I traveled around the world, I was diagnosed with bowel cancer three times and now the disease is terminal," he cried. I watched as He cried whilst having the shower. "Well if you need anything at all or any support please let me know," I murmured. It was then that I saw the true aspect of being a nurse and supporting patients at their darkest moments. Suddenly I heard a loud scream, and as I looked on the bathroom floor, I realized that the water from the shower had created a flood.

After the flood, Lucy called me to observe her putting a dressing on Clive. Lucy explained that Clive's dementia condition had escalated, and he was unaware of time or place. I watched as he lay in the bed as Lucy applied the honey dressing. "Who are you? I'm Hannah" I replied

"Is that your mother?" he shouted looking at Lucy. "No Lucy is your nurse," I replied. I was so unskilled in my communication technique. I gently picked up his war medal from the table. Suddenly Clive snatched the medal, angrily from my hand. "Give that back to you thieving bitch!" he scowled. It was then that Clive pushed Lucy away, I felt like I was a hindrance, I felt like my skills were underdeveloped.

In the afternoon Lucy allowed me to take the observations of the patients. It took me ten minutes to take the observations, I was so nervous about making a mistake. I completed Simon's observations and watched as his wife sat beside me. "Goodness me, the staff are looking younger than ever, how old are you darling?"

"Eighteen," I muttered.

"She is just a student nurse darling, loves to talk, it appears, " Simon groaned. I felt so belittled in their presence I felt like everything I did was wrong and judged.

I enjoyed my break. It was a great time to relax and reflect on the morning's events. I spent my time drinking my Ribena and consuming my cheese and crackers. After I arrived back in the ward, I noticed Richard sitting in his chair crying, looking like he had given up.

"What is wrong Richard?" I asked.

"I just spoke to the social worker, and I just discovered that my house will be taken away from me, they say it's inhabitable and not safe." Richard cried, wiping the tears from his eyes. I wanted to help him, to complete a small act to support him. I offered to help shave his beard and help him with a bedside wash, which he had continuously refused.

I was equipped with scissors, a bowl of warm water, and shaving foam. As I slowly moved his dirty top uncovered in dog hair and food stains. I found myself holding my breath, but this was the essence of being a nurse, accepting patients unconditionally.

I began to cut through Richard's beard with the razor-sharp scissors, and helped him to wash his dirty fingernails, and applied deodorant towards him, and I then helped him to put on his brand-new checkered suit. I watched as Richard sat in his brand-new outfit, and he looked up at me and smiled. "You have made me feel so much better," he smiled.

It was then that Trudy and Ann ordered me to help them from behind the curtain of Donald's bed space, to help him to freshen up and assist him back into the chair, as he required hoisting in the afternoon due to a decrease in his mobility. Ann and Trudy looked so alike, they were five foot one and they both had their hair in bunches, and always stood defiantly with their fists clenched. "Can you help us assist Donald back into his bed?" Ann asked.

I watched as a distressed Donald sat uncomfortably in the recliner chair. I could feel Ann and Trudy's eyes bore into me, as I placed the hoist straps around me, and we assisted Donald into his bed. Donald became increasingly agitated as he began to kick and punch out, as we attempted him to settle in the bed. Donald grabbed items from his table and began to throw them angrily on the floor including his jug of water causing a river to form on the floor. I witnessed the challenges of supporting patients with dementia in the hospital and could see that the noise, lighting, and change in the environment deeply affected them.

 I witnessed first-hand how busy the life of a nurse was in the ward. I watched as she ran around, completing notes, talking to family members, completing drug rounds, and liaising with various members of the multidisciplinary team. I felt overwhelmed. I wondered how I could survive working on the frontline for twelve hours each day.

It was then that Lucy ushered me over towards her as she sat at the Nurse's desk. "Kate, our next task is quite difficult. I have just spoken to the ward consultant Dr. Quatzy, he has provided us with Clive's latest scan results, and it shows that his illness has progressed, and he now only has less than a month to live," she sighed.

I looked on in sadness as I observed Clive's granddaughter skipping around his bed, holding up a rainbow picture in his hand, whilst his distraught daughter held onto his hand. We walked up nervously to Clive's bed space, with Dr. Quatzy, the health care assistant guided his Granddaughter to the playroom so that the news could be delivered.

I watched as Dr. Quatzy lowered his black-rimmed glasses and held onto his board.

"I'm sorry to tell you Clive but the results from your latest scan have shown that the cancer has spread, and we have now found multiple nodules on the lung."

We watched as Dr. Quatzy walked away with his clipboard as Clive collapsed into the bed in a flood of tears.

"Please Clive, you must not get upset, we are all here for you, let me make you both a cup of tea, and we can talk about options," Lucy smiled. I watched as Clive and his daughter shared a private embrace, trying to comprehend the devastating news.

I watched as Lucy walked into the kitchen and she broke down into a flood of tears. Lucy had looked after Clive for over a month on the ward, and had built a connection with Clive and his family.

I felt through the shift that I was following Lucy around, I was so nervous and lacked the skills needed to communicate with patients with complex needs. Lucy appeared to be working to a strict regime, she completed two drugs rounds, multiple ward rounds, and spent a long period of time completing care round notes.

I felt a warm and welcoming feeling from the staff on the ward round, the The ward manager and senior staff would constantly ask how I was and offered to answer any questions. The ward manager organized two staff huddles during the shift, which included a time to talk about the changes in the ward. The manager offered us tea, cakes, and biscuits, which helped us all feel refreshed. The ward manager had a strong sense of staff wellbeing, and ensured that each member of staff was happy and supported throughout the shift.

At the end of the shift, I was exhausted and as I arrived home, I quickly consumed my home-baked pizza, before collapsing onto the sofa in an extreme state of exhaustion.

The next morning, I work up to multiple social media posts of my friends back home in the US. Many were enjoying the fun of their Arts degrees with three-hour lectures per week and constant partying. As a nursing student, I felt like I spent my days off completing my essays and the remainder of my time was spent completing nursing practice. I observed my best friend Arlena partying at a beach with the first-year students, and sitting with her friends on the beautiful lawns on the grounds of Harvard University. Whilst I was completing a high intense placement on a twelve-hour shift, trying hard to soak up the atmosphere of the ward.

Chapter 2 A baby is born!

I was apprehensive for my first night, I had never stayed up all night before, I was worried there would be little for me to do, I was worried about making a mistake. I packed my satchel with crackers and cheese, chocolate to try and keep me awake. I also packed a toothbrush and a radio to use on my break. Nothing could prepare me for what I was about to encounter on the night shift.

I walked down the long country road and followed the light of the full moon towards the hospital. I once heard that on the night of a full moon strange events occur. I was calm and felt prepared for the shift, knowing that Lucy was always on hand to support me.

As I walked onto the ward that evening I was struck by the calm atmosphere, the flickering lights from the patient's side lamps, and the dull beeping sound coming from the intravenous machines. In the Handover room was Lucy, Alberta, a sixty-nine-year-old nurse with over forty-seven years of experience, Jonathan a senior nurse who despised students and an agency nurse called Angel, and she truly was an angel.

The healthcare assistants on the shift were Samantha Richards, Samantha had over thirty years of experience, and Sylvia Buns, a sixty-five-year-old woman from Bulgaria who was very eccentric, but very caring, and overly affectionate to her staff members.

As we finished the handover, Sylvia asked me to go to the laundry closet with her to collect the blankets and sheets for the night

Shift. I walked to the laundry cupboard, and as I opened the door, I could hear a banging noise against the wall, a hand banging against the door, and a faint cry for help. I took a deep breath, and believed that the noises were just the cries of patients in another ward. Then I could hear the bang against the wall again and a stronger cry shout for help. I rushed out of the room, and behind the closet were the public toilets in the corridor. I quickly rushed into the toilets and there she was to my complete horror laying down in the cubicle toilet was a lady laying on the floor in labor. She lay in her blue hospital gown, her face dripping in sweat, I looked at the fear in her face, the expression of fear on her face.

"Oh nurse, I'm so happy you're here!" She gasped. I could feel my hands trembling as I noticed the emergency buzzer was out of order. I stood up in a panic, "I need to go and get help for you, -"
"No, you can't leave me please," she yelled. I had to trust my instinct. I realized the woman was hysterical and she needed urgent help. I ran out to the derelict gloomy hospital corridor, and there was Sylvia.
"Sylvia, there's a lady in labor in the bathroom," I gasped. Suddenly Sylvia charged down the corridor, and walked into the bathroom, "My Goodness got towels and turned the tap on," Sylv pleaded.
"We need to call for help!"

"No, I trained as a midwife in Bulgaria, I know what to do and it's too late to call for help!" she smiled.

I quickly ran out and panicked turning on the taps and grabbing the sheets and hot towels from the laundry. I quickly ran back into the bathroom and quickly played the towels and sheets around the floor. The lady grabbed my hand tightly, as she began to scream. My heart felt as if it was going to explode out of my chest. I was petrified, a first-year nursing student faced my first medical emergency and I felt so lost.

"I'm going to die," the lady cried. "What's your name?"

"Daphne," she replied.

"Daphne, just breathe," I yelled as she gripped more tightly onto my hand, as sweat poured from her brow.

I nervously gazed at Sylvia as she kneeled in front of Daphne.

"The baby is coming with just one push; you can do it!" Sylvia yelled.

I watched as Daphne took several deep breaths, her face filled with fear, I felt my mind freezing in shock, I began to feel like my hand was going to collapse. We had only been in the room for half an hour, but I felt like we were frozen in time.

"Just one final push and you are there, Daphne," Sylv beamed. I watched as Daphne took one final push, and moments later Sylv presented me with a baby boy, wrapped in a blue blanket. Sylv had washed the blood off his face and passed him towards Daphne. I watched as Daphne began to cry, overwhelmed with emotion.

"Thank you both, so much, both of you have made such a difference, he is perfect," She beamed. I felt so overwhelmed to be part of such a private and important moment in Daphne's life.

"Right now, you can call for help," Sylvia smiled. I looked at Sylvia in complete disbelief. I quickly rushed to the ward and alerted the doctors and nurses, and my mentor Lucy looked at me in shock.

"My goodness are you ok? I'm in shock, you did so well," Lucy beamed.

Daphne and her baby boy were quickly taken to the neonatal ward where they both received medical attention. Later that day, along with Sylvia, we were ordered to the neonatal ward, and our photo was taken which I later discovered in the national process. It was a moment I will never forget, I had never expected to have been part of the emergency.

Once I returned to the ward, after the emergency, Lucy gave me an hour's break to reflect on what happened and to calm my nerves. I soon realized how working on the night shift was so different from the day shift. The patient's observations were taken at 9 pm, whilst the next set would be taken at 6 am in the morning. Certain patients would require medication or assistance to the ward, but most of the night I spent with Lucy monitoring the patients and talking through the nursing observations. As I walked into my bay, I could hear Richard whispering to me. "Anna How are you? It's great to see you," He smiled.

I observed Richard sitting up in the bed he was wearing his blue-striped pajamas and next to him were his bags packed. I could see how positive and happy he was. "Anna I want to thank you so much for helping me with the wash, I feel so much more content, the social services have offered me temporary accommodation and a support worker, you and Lucy have really supported me!" Richard smiled. It felt great to have made a difference in Richard's life, to see him gain his confidence and independence. This was the true essence of being a nurse, helping the most vulnerable people in society, and helping patients in their darkest moments.

I then walked over to Simon the 'strict headteacher' to take his blood sugar reading. "Simon please can I take your blood sugar reading?"
Suddenly his face began to boil red with anger. "Excuse me I was just in the middle of deep sleep. How dare you!" he roared. I soon realized I could not please all patients and that I would need to become more resilient to the patient's moods. I took Simon's blood sugar and he tucked himself back under the covers.

Mark, the patient being monitored by a mental health nurse, was spending his final night on the ward, before being moved to a psychiatric hospital, due to a deterioration in his mental health condition. As part of Adult nursing, mental health was not touched on in great depth, so most of my experience with mental health was based on the job training.

I observed Clive in the bed, sleeping, he was now on continuous morphine, and able to sleep during the night.

As I sat at the nurse's station, I went through my student nurse booklet and revised the key anatomy that I needed to progress. After one hour I heard a loud thud in the bay, it was Donald. Donald was living with sundowning, a part of his dementia illness in which he was unable to distinguish between night and day. Donald charged towards the nurse's station and stamped his hand on the nurse's station.

"I want to go home; my mother is expecting me home. I should have been home at ten."

"Why don't you accompany Donald on a walk," Lucy offered.

I walked with Donald slowly up and down the corridor, suggesting for him to sit down and take a rest break, when I should have been encouraging him to walk along the corridor based on his own free will. As part of the dementia condition, a person's memory can refresh back to their childhood. In Donald's current state of mind, he believed that he was fifteen years ago, and needed to return to his mother's house. I observed his deep confusion, believing the staffroom was a restroom and mistaking a buzzer noise like the sound of an incoming train.

As we reached the door, I wrongfully stood in front of the door, explaining to Donald that it was locked.

"Move, I want to go home, I need you to move please," He warned.

"It's really late Donald, would you like to sit in your chair, and I can make you a cup of tea?" I offered. I watched as Donald's face began to fill red with rage, he grabbed his stick in his hand and went to hit me, "Get out of the way, now!" he screamed. Donald then began to knock on the door with the walking stick eventually causing a huge dent on the door.

It was then that I observed Sylvia take Donald by the hand and she guided him to the bed. I watched as Sylvia took a gentle turn to support Donald, and she provided a table and chair for Donald to keep him stimulated whilst he was awake. There was so much I needed to learn about dementia, and I realized how inexperienced I was.

Throughout the night shift, Lucy discussed some common drugs used in the ward, and presented me with an anatomy picture book to complete, to help aid my understanding. The remainder of the night shift involved measuring the fluid and urine output of the patients and filling in the patient's care plans and notes. I felt so exhausted during the night shift, I overloaded myself with chocolates and carbohydrates, which managed to give me the energy I needed to complete the shift.

My first placement was filled with so many challenges which I felt were based around my lack of experience, and my underdeveloped communication skills in supporting patients with complex needs.

The support from my mentor Lucy was invaluable, through watching her practice, I learned the true essence of kindness and compassion. Lucy was very kind and gentle, and would get to know all her patients supporting the patient's physical and mental needs. As part of my first placement, I learned the basics of nursing care such as providing personal care to patients, completing baseline results, and following clinical guidelines based on the patient's clinical results.

Lucy always had time for me as a student, and would always answer any questions and help me with any queries I had. At times Lucy would test me on my knowledge and I would then become aware of gaps in my knowledge. I soon realized during my first placement that no books, videos, or tutorials could teach me how to be a nurse.

After my first placement, I had a few months gap between my next placement, and a shocking discovery in the loft of my Grandmother's house left me shaken. It was October 1st, and I decided to explore further into the house and did not realize that I was about to discover a secret family revelation. In the boxes, in the loft, I discovered more pictures of her during her work as a stunt woman, but the box full of her diary entries suggested to me that she had many secrets, and a hidden life that she fought hard to keep away from others.

In the boxes, I discovered her diary which included extracts from her life as a stunt woman over her forty-year career. Behind her glamorous lifestyle, was a secret battle with depression, an eating disorder, and deep-rooted self-esteem issues. My Grandmother revealed in her diary extracts that she was deeply distressed from newspaper articles which criticized her weight. As I read further into my Grandmother's diary extracts I was shocked to discover that at the age of twenty-five, after the passing of her parents in a car accident, she made the shocking discovery that she was adopted, and found that her biological parents lived in Buckinghamshire in London. My Grandmother discovered that her mother gave birth to her when she was sixteen and was forced to adopt her. She then discovered that her parents became successful journalists, and published a successful magazine reaching thousands of readers. On her 27th birthday, my Grandma traveled to London to track down her parents, when she reached the house, she saw that her parents lived in a grand mansion. She discovered she had two brothers and a sister. When she spoke to her mother, she marveled at her beauty, as she sat in her pink sequined dress and her blonde hair was wrapped neatly in a bun. However, Anita was devastated to discover that her adoptive mother did not want her to be part of the family and expressed that she was a symbol of shame from her past. My Grandmother expressed in the diary extract that she never revealed that she was adopted to another person.

It was then that I realized I had a big decision to make to keep my Grandmother's secret heartache a secret or reveal what I discovered to my own family.

Chapter 3: The community experience

My second placement was in a community district nurse setting, and as part of the experience, I managed to treat patients from a range of backgrounds and life experiences, and to see what life is like for patients in their day to day life. As I walked into the district nurse office, I felt so relaxed and calm, there were no sirens, shouts for help, or people running around. The district nurse office was filled with a range of health professionals, such as Nurses, Doctors, and physiotherapy and occupational health teams. My mentor, Mags, was very different from my first mentor Lucy. Mags was very outspoken, straight speaking, and treated nursing as a task-orientated job. Mags was fifty-five, with wild curly black hair wrapped up in a beehive style. Mags was a chronic smoker and would often smoke over fifty cigarettes a day.

"Hi, I'm Mags, what's your name?"

"Hannah from California,"

"Oh, a yank,"

"An American," I replied.

"Well this is the office, we complete our notes here, from 9-2 we visit patients, we arrive back at the office at half 2 and once we complete notes you can go at half four," She explained.

That morning I entered Mag's mini convertible, as I stepped in, I could smell the deep stench of smoke filling the air in the care. I felt consumed in smoke I could not breathe. I sat in the car, in shock as Mag's blasted the greatest hits of meatloaf from her radio, I felt like my eardrums were going to burst. I felt nervous as a student, throughout my life I found it hard to settle into new environments, and as a student nurse, I had to adapt quickly to new environments and work around my new mentors.

On my first day, Mags presented me with a list of over ten patients we were due to see, and we had several tasks to complete ranging from taking observations, to completing dressings, to providing end-of-life care. The first house we arrived at was of an eighty-nine-year-old lady named June who was living with dementia. June was found wandering in the streets and was admitted to the hospital where she was later diagnosed with dementia. June's only daughter lived in America, but their severed relationship meant that they did not keep in touch.

June's house was a spectacular Edwardian style house, with a ten-acre garden. Our visit to June was a follow-up visit to assess how well she was managing at home, and to assess if she required any more care.

June greeted us at the door dressed in a blue dressing-gown, her blonde curly hair was hidden under her silk red hat.

"So wonderful to see you both, come in, come in," she smiled. As we stepped inside the house, I could smell the stench of rotten vegetables and animal feces. June guided us into the living room, which was covered in Elvis memorabilia, on the walls were pictures of Elvis throughout his career and on her radio, she blasted the greatest hits of Elvis.

As I sat down, June sat closely next to me and began to pull my cheeks with her hands, "Isn't she lovely, she has a lovely fat face, like Susan Boyle," she giggled. It was then that June held onto my hand as Mag's before her assessment, taking June's vital observations including her blood pressure and temperature, which were all in the normal parameters. "How have you been since your hospital admission, how have you found being at home?" Mag's asked.

"It's ok it can be very lonely at times, some days I have no one to speak to, I miss my parents. I am always losing my notebook where I write my appointment reminders. I feel quite depressed at times because I can't do the tasks I used to, I struggle with cooking," she exclaimed.

"Do you mind if we can have a look around your house?" Mags asked.

Then we followed Mag's around the house, and we looked around in shock as she guided us around the house. The kitchen was filthy with two scrawny cats crawling around the work surfaces. Crushed biscuits and litter were scattered all over the floor. Inside the fridge the bread was covered in green mold, the half-eaten pasta bake was swarming with maggots. As we walked around the house, we witnessed feces on the floor in the toilets and a stale smell of rotting cabbage. It was clear to see that June was struggling in her home and she required urgent intervention.

After looking around upstairs we returned downstairs to the living room, and June began singing, 'devil in disguise' by Elvis.

"June, it really has been lovely to see you today, but after looking around your house we feel you may need more support."

"No, I'm ok, I have Elvis, I have my songs, I'm not going into care," she demanded. It was then that June went to the kitchen to make us a cup of tea with the sour milk, which we gently refused.
I looked at June as she looked at me with tears in her eyes, "I'm going to be ok darling? Promise me" she smiled.

I held onto June's hand gently, "don't worry June we are going to help you," I smiled. It was then that I exited the house and as we sat in the car, I watched as the mask of June's tough exterior began to crumble, and a single tear fell from her cheek. Mag's called the social services and the mental health assessment team, requesting an urgent assessment. June presented as a vulnerable adult and required urgent help. June was later assessed by the social services and was sectioned under the mental health act. I was happy that day that we could help June, I felt empowered as a student nurse that I could help her.

We then visited our next patient's house, Greg, a forty-year-old man with chronic arthritis and type 2 diabetes. Greg lived on the top floor of the apartment complex, and required his dressings to be changed. "Now you must be careful Ana Greg is a very cantankerous man, he may not let you perform the dressing. Greg is living with Bipolar disorder and he may display unusual behavior, but above all remain calm." Mags warned. As I entered Greg's flat, I observed him laying across the couch, watching the Texas chainsaw massacre. Greg was over twenty-five stones and sat with the porridge and jam in his hand.

"Who the fuck is she?" he scowled.

"This is Hannah she is from California, she is a first-year student nurse and she has come to complete your dressings today if that's ok?" Mags replied.

"I suppose so, but I don't want a fucking yank messing up my dressing and then I will get an infection!" he scowled.

I was nervous as I completed the dressing as my hands started to tremble, I observed as Greg's anger began to turn red as I patted the dressing down. "You fucking fat, ugly, bitch you have put it on wrong!" He shouted. It was then that he grabbed onto my arms and I gasped in shock, before Mag's stepped in, "No she has completed the dressing correctly, try and remain calm." Mag's warned.

I slowly stepped back from an Angry Greg, as he took a few deep breaths and regained his composure.

Within five minutes he was smiling whilst continuing to watch his film.

"Thank you nurses for your help!" he beamed.

It was interesting to see how Greg's behavior and demeanor could change within minutes. As staff working on the frontline in the NHS, we had to be resilient against the aggressive behavior of our patients.

I nearly suffocated as I traveled back in the car with Mag's. She continued to smoke rapidly as we sped down the motorway. The next patient was Violet, a sixty-eight-year-old woman living with exacerbation with her COPD, and had just been diagnosed with stage three lung cancer, our reason to visit Violet was to discuss treatment plans. Violet lived in a two-bedroomed bungalow which she shared with her husband Mike who died the previous year. As we reached the door, Violet stood wearing a smart pea-green suit, her blonde hair was Curly and wrapped neatly in a bun. Violet ushered us into the house, and we sat on the leather couch and drank the cup of tea from the bluebird cups.

"So Violet, this is Hannah, a student from California, she is in her first year."

"Oh, Hannah you are so pretty, both me and Mike visited Vegas and California back in 1972 on our honeymoon, you are so lucky to have lived there," Violet explained.

It was then that Violet's Alsatian dog sat next to her on the couch. I could feel his eyes bore into mine, I was terrified of dog's and felt extremely uncomfortable. My face and legs turned red and I developed a nervous rash.

"Well, Violet as you're aware we are here today to discuss your decision regarding treatment plans."

I watched as Violet's hands began to shake, "I've given it some thought, and I have decided against any treatment. Mag's if my time is up it's up, I do not want to be a burden to my daughter, she had to look after Mike when he fell ill and she can't go through it again, I don't want to go through it." she cried. I could see Mag's stir in Shock at Violet's admission, but as nurses, we had to respect violet's free will and not influence her in any decisions.

"I understand this must be a difficult situation for you but please find the number for Macmillan cancer support in the booklet I have here, and if you need time to talk through options we are always here for you," Mags assured her. Violet moved towards Mags and embraced her, "Thank you both for your support. I will consider my options." Violet smiled.

It was then that I took Violet's observations, noticing that her respiration rate was high due to the COPD condition. Every breath Violet took was a struggle, her lungs were affected by the amount of smoke she had consumed since she was sixteen.

We carried on our journey to the final house, a seventy-nine-year-old lady called Alina who was at the end stage of her liver cancer condition. Aline lived in a grand three-story mansion in the heart of Camden. We drove up the long stone pathway to the house, which was hidden behind several oak trees. As we made our way into the house, we stood in the hallway, in which the golden staircase was situated which led to the ten-bedroom upstairs. The windows in the mansion were stained windows of the famous works of Pablo Picasso. We walked up the spiral staircase, and followed the red carpet to Alina's bedroom, the grandest room in the house. Alina previously worked as a musical theatre director and owned three musical schools in England. Alina's bedroom was thrilled with pictures of her directing various theatre shows throughout her forty-year career. The window of Alina's room overlooked her ten-acre garden. I observed Alina laying in her huge king size bed, she appeared to disappear under the sheets.

Alina began to sing in her bed along to Enya 'sail away' as it played on her cd player. Alina was in good spirits despite living with a terminal illness.

"How have you been?" Mags asked.

"I've had a great weekend, I watched my favorite film 'gone with the wind' and I finished knitting my Granddaughters birthday clothes. Tomorrow I am holding a dinner party in my room, with a few of my previous classmates from the theatre school. "

I then observed Mag's administering the medication, with care and patience. Alina's end of life medication was delivered through a syringe driver.

"How is your mobility Alina? How have you been sleeping recently?" Mag's asked.

"I can walk to and from the bathroom, and the carers are a great support in helping me to dress in the mornings. I am more tired and tend to nap during the day," she explained. I sat next to Alina and helped to position her in the bed ready for her lunch. It was then that Alina discussed her career in theatre, training thousands of students to achieve their dreams in musical theatre. I admired Alina's strength and positivity despite her illness, she was able to enjoy her hobbies.

After visiting Alina, we made our way back to the office, and I felt like I was suffocating as Mag's consumed up to five cigarettes on the journey back.

As we arrived back at the office, I devoured my cheese sandwich and Yorkshire tea. I then assisted Mags with completing the patient notes. My placement in the community setting was very different from hospital placement. In the community setting, I was able to observe the private life of patients and to see the impact of the home environment on the mental and physical wellbeing of patients. Whilst much of my community placement was devoid of direct nursing skills, I developed my communication and problem-solving skills. Whilst nurses had high demands in the hospital environment, I observed demands in the community, such as getting through the caseload of patients in a day,

Mag was a very caring nurse, and I learned so much from her as a mentor, in terms of the theory behind nursing skills and I learned how to treat the whole person, not just the condition. In the community, I felt there was more time to talk through my nursing observations in a calm and relaxed environment.

After the placement, I decided I wanted to find out more about my Grandmother's biological history, and decided to visit the house of my biological great Grandparents, to see if any surviving members of her family were living in the house. I was nervous at visiting the house, knowing that my own mother was unaware of the secret life. I walked up to the thatched Edwardian cottage, my hands were trembling, and my heart began to beat faster. I knocked on the door and an elderly lady in her eighties opened the door. The elderly lady stood in her emerald sequin dress, her blonde hair was hidden under a blue flat cap, her eyes were a brilliant blue. The elderly lady resembled my Grandma, she was my great aunt Imelda.

"Hello, I'm looking for a member of the Smith family, my Grandmother came visiting this house over twenty years ago but-"

"Agatha? Are you related to Agatha? Please come in," Imelda whispered, her hands were trembling. I sat in the dining room, and Imelda brought me a cream scone and a green tea.

"My mother told me everything about Agatha just before she died. Mum gave birth to Agatha at sixteen years of age, but her parents were devout Catholics, and she was forced to have the baby in secret and later was forced to give her up for adoption." Imelda claimed

"Gran went to look for them. Why did your parents abandon her again?"

"Mum could never get over the emotional trauma of Agatha, and it was a part of her life she was trying hard to forget, she could never accept Agatha as her daughter," Imelda added.

"You seem to have had a good life, I can see your graduation picture from medical school, you seem to be doing well, my Grandmother was innocent in all of this," I explained.

I could see how uncomfortable Imelda was whilst talking to me, and I soon realized it was a mistake trying to discover my family secret.

I quickly jumped up from the couch and began to run out of the house.

"Please don't go under these circumstances!" Imelda shouted.

I later wished that I didn't explore my biological family, and soon realized that it was a big mistake. I decided it was best to keep my Grandmother's letters hidden from my Mother. My time in London as a student nurse and living on my own was very hard at times. After an emotionally distressing shift, I did not have anyone to confide in, and a long-distance phone call did not help me.

On my day off I would spend my time reading, dancing, and getting involved in sports at the university, such as badminton and cross country running. After My community placement, I was placed in a range of different settings including a stroke ward, a theatre placement, and a busy sixty bedded orthopedic ward. I worked so hard to complete my academic essays, but balancing theory work with twelve-hour shifts was particularly stressful.

Chapter 4: The final battle

My final placement was on a general medical ward, in a small community placement. As it was my management placement, I had to prove that I was competent to work as a nurse and to complete tasks confidently without direct nursing supervision.

My mentor Brian was the difficult mentor I was yet to meet. As soon as I met Brian, he stated that I had to be a very good student if I was to pass under his mentorship. Later that day I could hear sighs and disapproving looks when the other staff discovered who my mentor was. I had a strong feeling that this was going to be a difficult placement.

I took the handover that morning on the ward and every staff member had a pleasant disposition except for Brian. Throughout the medication round, I was asked a series of rigorous nursing questions, but I passed everyone, I felt as If Brian was attempting to catch me out. It was then that Brian sat at his desk in our bay, he sat inpatient with his arms folded.

"I will be watching you from afar, I want to see how well you manage caring for a bay on your own.

On my first shift, I had to support patients with complex needs, and I was working with a health care assistant called Trudy. Trudy would constantly leave the ward for a cigarette and was often found on her mobile phone. The first Patient was John, a fifty-eight-year-old man, admitted due to pains in his chest, and later had triple bypass surgery and he was awaiting his medications to go home, waiting impatiently.

The second patient was Martin, an eighty-one-year man with Lewy bodies dementia admitted following a worsening of his dementia condition. John required one on one supervision, and I fought hard for Trudy to sit with him, at times when I had to leave the bay.

The third patient was Dean, a fifty-five-year-old man admitted following a change in his diabetes condition and was awaiting a review by a specialist diabetic nurse.

The fourth patient was Sean a sixty-seven-year-old man who was over twenty stone and was admitted following self-neglect, he was found with multiple pressure sores on his body, and he required multiple redressing every day.

The Final patient was Gurajeevan, a sixty-year-old man from Bangladesh admitted with a chest infection. Guajeevan could not speak any English, which made care and his demands very difficult.

  I helped the patients with their washes with Trudy whilst Brian mysteriously disappeared.

Martin was very angry during the wash after initially being relaxed. "Martin I am trying to help you with your wash," I offered. Martin went to punch me in the face narrowingly missing my face. "You bastard American, you keep away from me," he shouted.

"Come on Martin after your wash we can go for a nice walk," Trudy offered. "Shut up your ugly fat cow!" he snapped. After a long struggle, we helped John to put on his pajamas. Being on a ward is so difficult for patients living with dementia, due to the noise, different people, and lack of good communication. I watched as Trudy walked with Martin to the day room, and I later observed her taking pictures of herself with her camera phone. I managed to finish washing the patients at 10 am, and I could feel the glare of Brian's eyes bore into me.

I had to complete Sean's dressings on his legs with the help of Brian in helping him to reposition in the bed. Sean appeared deeply depressed and every time I attempted to engage in conversation, he would ignore me. I thought about the best type of interventions for him, including talking therapies and counseling. I quickly realized that the mental health services with long waiting times had a big impact on patients. Sean was referred to a mental health group but had to wait three months after his referral for it to start. In this time period, he had made two suicide attempts with no interim support. "Do you have any family support Sean?" I asked.

"Stop with the chit chat and carry on with the dressing," Brian moaned.

I felt like a child, I felt angry that Brian was avoiding communication and saw nursing only as a process.

"Where are my medications, I've been waiting for ages!" John yelled.

"I will check now," I promised. I left the bay and enquired with the pharmacist department about the arrival of the medication but was told that there was a long waiting list.

I felt relaxed when the brain was on his break, and I completed the observations, blood sugars, and patients care plans, making sure that I kept them up to date. As I spoke to Dean, he revealed to me my worst thoughts. "You need to watch out for that Brian guy, he dislikes students, he gave the last student nurse hell, he made her cry, and she was only doing her best. You need to speak up" he warned. I smiled, nervously, surprised at how accurate Dean was and I knew how vulnerable I was.

It was then that Trudy walked back with Martin, as he began to feel tired and he rested on his bed.

I watched as Trudy sat in her chair texting. "Trudy, can you help me fill in the care plans?

"Later" she shot back.

"Now" I replied.

"No later." she shot back. It was true that as a student it was sometimes more difficult to manage the staff than the patients.

I worked so hard on the ward, and I watched as Brian performed the qualified nurse duties, such as administering the controlled drugs and intravenous medication. I was unaware that he was about to erupt and squash all my efforts.

Gurajeevans wife appeared wearing a red pajama suit, her curly black hair reached the floor. She applied Guajeevan with multiple colorful blankets. It was then that Gurajeevan's wife began to shout, "He needs more watchers, my husband needs biscuits and treats, we need extra pillows." It was then that I watched as Gurajeevan's wife spilt the water jug all over the floor and knocked the contents off his table and onto the floor. I felt so exhausted. Just before my shift ended, Brain ushered me into the office. "How do you think you did today?" he asked.

"Well, I've tried so hard," I responded. I watched as his false smile turned to anguish.

"I felt you took your time to complete the observations, you responded slowly to Gurajeevans wife, you came back one minute after your lunch break. It was a really bad first day" He muttered. I felt so tired after being on my feet all day, and I was given no recognition. I drove home that night and collapsed onto my bed in a flood of tears.

I struggled with Brian as my mentor until I felt like I could no longer function in the ward as a student nurse. Every day I was constantly belittled, bullied, and humiliated by Brian. I would feel sick going to work, and instead of feeling like a student, I felt like a nurse who required persecution.

After a particularly stressful shift I felt so upset, that I collapsed into a heap onto the floor in the sluice, and the sister in the ward Jean discovered me and ushered me into her office.

"Goodness what is the matter tells me all about it?" she began.

"I can't cope here, I feel like leaving, I am constantly bullied and humiliated." I cried.

It was then that Jean held onto my hand tenderly, "Brian is on annual leave next week, I will be taking over your mentorship from now on, you will never work a shift with him again." She promised.

I felt relieved, I was almost ready to leave the setting, but Jean's supportive comments made me realize that help was available and that I was not on my own. It took just one act of kindness to help me realize I was not alone. In the following few weeks, I received so much support from Jane, I was tested in a calm relaxed environment, and I gained confidence in my management skills.

At the start of my final shift, I felt nervous and apprehensive, it was my final shift as a student nurse, and I had to prove I was competent to manage the ward without supervision, Jane would act as my 'observer' during the shift. After the handover, I had to allocate the nurses to their bay. I was working with Anita and Mary, they had both worked as nurses for over twenty years and were very supportive of me.

Then walked into my bay to meet my patients. The first patients were Ethel, a 99-year-old former veterinary surgeon who was admitted with confusion and was due to be assessed by the mental health team. Ethel required continuous supervision, so I ensured that the healthcare assistant Hayley supervised her. The second patient was Shelley, a seventy-two-year-old lady with dementia, Shelley was admitted due to the care home's inability to cope with her erratic behavior. The third patient was Kate, a ninety-year-old lady with end-stage dementia requiring end of life care support. Whilst the final patient was Harriet, Harriet was admitted due to an exacerbation in her MS condition.

I completed the medication rounds and the healthcare assistant Janet helped me set the patients up for washes whilst June assisted her. It was then that Dr. Harold the consultant arrived and as we completed the ward round, I was met with so many questions, "What was the physiotherapist review?" "How is the patient managing with eating and drinking?" I found myself constantly checking the notes on my handover sheet, but I answered the questions.

As I returned to my bay, chaos ensued, Janet was struggling in managing Ethel's behavior as she began to hit out. I walked over to quickly intervene.
"What's wrong?" I asked
"This lady here is keeping me hostage, I have a meeting with a senior veterinary surgeon at 11 pm." She stammered.
Following on from my experience of supporting patients with dementia, I could see that Ethel was bored and I wanted to encourage her to participate in purposeful activities. I walked with Ethel and Janet to the nursing station. I helped Ethel to sit down by the ward Clark at the nurse's station, and gave her a folder of paper, and encouraged her to file the paper into the poly pockets. Ethel was content sitting at the desk and felt like she had a purpose and was more relaxed.

It was then that I heard a shrill scream in the bay. Shelly had thrown her Zimmer frame against the wall. "Shelley what is wrong is there any way that I can help you," I asked.

"Get that man away from me, claiming to be my husband, get him away from me!" She shouted. I observed Shelley's husband crying at her bedside, feeling a sense of helplessness. I alerted June to ring a member of the raid assessment team, the mental health team to assess her immediately before her behavior escalated. I helped June to settle on the bed, and suddenly in a fit of rage she grabbed the water jug and threw the water all over me

"You silly bitch, get me out of here get me home!" she shouted. Finally, the rapid assessment team arrived, and they pulled the curtains around so that they could assess June.

I then assisted Kate with her fortisip drink, and together with June, we helped to reposition Kate. As Kate was at the end stage of her dementia condition, she needed to be repositioned every two hours, in order to prevent pressure sores. Kate was unable to communicate but found enjoyment in listening to her music on her cassette player.

After I repositioned Kate, I had to assist the porter in finding an oxygen cylinder to accompany Harriet to the Ct scan.

I felt like my head was about to spin, I had so many tasks to complete, I had to oversee the general management of the ward whilst updating the care plans, delegating tasks, and talking to relatives. As we had a staff member sick I had to assist Mary and Anita with their patient care rounds. I had watched how busy Anita was in her bay, whilst her shy first-year student Lisa appeared to trail behind her, and I witnessed Lisa spending more time with the healthcare assistants on the ward, as Anita presented a very hostile demeanor. As I walked up to the staffroom at lunchtime, I could hear Anita consulting with Mary about the difficulties she had as a mentor.

"I am really struggling with Lisa; she may be the first student I fail, and she is only in her first year."

"At least give her a chance, see how the next two weeks ago," Anita explained.

"Since she has started on the ward, she will not ask questions, she is turning up late and constantly taking extended breaks, I will have no choice but to fail her," she exclaimed.

I wanted to help Lisa in any way I could, failing her first year would have devastating consequences on her future career. I met with Lisa in the Nurse's office and offered my phone number and email, explaining that I would help her in any way I could, to prevent her from falling. As I was nearing the end of my student nurse journey, I felt an overwhelming need to support other student nurses.

I returned to my bay that afternoon and went behind the curtain in Kate's bed space and had sadly discovered that she had passed away. Kate 's family had spent hours with her and in the short interval that they left she passed. In a way, I felt comforted knowing that she was now no longer in discomfort. I looked around the pictures of her placed on the wall, including a picture of her in her Doctor's coat on a ward in London, whilst another picture showed her standing with her family holding an award for outstanding achievement for over fifty years in the NHS. "Thank you, Kate, for helping so many patients, you truly have lived a wonderful life," I began. I then worked together with Jean to complete the last offices. When Kate's daughter arrived, I guided her into the relatives' room, and when I gave her the news, she broke down in a flood of tears.

In the afternoon I completed my final medication round, and June took me to the office. I was shaking and trembling as I entered, and as I sat at the table, I saw a sponge cake with 'congratulations Hannah' scrawled in white vanilla icing.

"Congratulations, you have passed. It has been wonderful working with you, and I feel that you will make an outstanding nurse. "Thank you so much for your support!" I smiled. It felt wonderful after three years, to have finally achieved my dream, whilst overcoming the obstacles, such as the difficult mentor Brian, and my constant struggle of juggling practical work with my university academic essays.

I changed throughout my career from a naive, shy nervous person, to a confident self-aware person. I had learned the true essence of how to provide safe and efficient care. I spent the next three months with my family in California unwinding, it felt therapeutic relaxing on the beach and resting my tired feet.

When I returned to the UK, I gained a position in a general medicine ward, and I have spent the past five years in the ward, and I am now a specialist Diabetic nurse. I never revealed the contents of my Grandmother's letters and kept my family secret hidden. The skills I feel are needed to be a student nurse are resilience, kindness, and compassion. I walked into nursing as a shy introverted young woman and left a different person.

Tom's Nursing journey

Chapter 5: New Beginnings

Many people believe that nursing is a vocation, a career they were born into. I always feel like I fell into my career as a nurse. I had spent so many years trying to find the perfect job, many of the jobs I undertook ended in a disaster. In my first job as a customer assistant in Marks and Spencer, I made countless mistakes, and then it ended in the ultimate disaster. I was asked to dress the mannequins in the shop window and accidentally dressed the female mannequins in men's suits which was the final straw. In my role in McDonald's I went into the lift and ended up in the rubbish tip covered in oil and waste. Then I worked on a nightline help service and fell asleep during the shift and woke up in the morning with the president of the student union giving me my final paycheck.

After a disastrous run of jobs in my late teens, I then gained a place on a politics degree at Oxford University. After three years I finished my degree, and I gained a job as a journalist at a local newspaper. Whilst I enjoyed my job, I felt like I was working in a toxic environment. I worked with colleagues who would step over you to get a promotion. My manager Clive was very strict and would seek out mistakes and would shout at the team members in front of colleagues. I would work hard every day meeting targets and meeting deadlines, but I never received any feedback or praise for my work.

I left my career as a journalist at the age of twenty-two. I wanted to help people, I wanted to make a difference. I watched an NHS recruitment video, and it struck a chord with me, watching the nurses supporting patients in the emergency department following a road traffic accident. I wanted to make a difference in the lives of vulnerable people, rather than spend my life behind a desk.

I lived with my parents in York, they both worked as Librarians in the local library, whilst my older brother Ben worked as an accountant at the world trade center in Birmingham. As the younger sibling, I always found myself catching up with my brother. I would spend day and night revising for an exam

And only just achieve a pass, whilst my brother would not revise but achieve full marks.

I was so nervous on my first day as a student nurse, I was terrified and apprehensive. I spent three months putting plasters on mannequins, learning skills in the clinical room, and sitting for hours in lectures learning the theory of nursing.

As I stepped outside I walked to the train station and the heavens opened, I was drenched in the torrential rain and shivered as I arrived on the old historic train, I wondered if the patients would like me, and I wondered if my mentor would be supportive to me as a person new to the care sector. Most of all I wanted to make a difference in the lives of the patients.

I was nervous as I entered the busy hospital in York, and I entered the busy thirty bedded medical wards. I stood in bewilderment as I watched the nurse's rising through the ward, taking observations, writing notes, assisting patients to the toilet, and updating care plans with ferocious speed. I felt like a child on my day of school, my hands were shaking, and I felt like my heart was ready to explode.

I walked into the handover room and saw the stern nurses waiting in the staffroom at the handover. My mentor Maureen sat looking bemused, her messy blonde hair was wrapped in a bun. The ward manager Anya refused to look at me as she buried her eyed in the handover sheet. The other nurse on shift Eunice arrived late and as she rushed to sit down, she knocked Maureen's tea over on the table. "Fuck sake, Eunice, be careful, Eunice!" Maureen yelled. The healthcare assistants Maria and Debra were polar opposites. Maria was bossy and would bark orders at students and staff. Debra was from London and was so approachable and would always make time for the patients.

As I stood outside after the handover, I saw my mentor Maureen look at me up and down in contempt, I got the impression she was being forced to mentor me. "Tom have you ever worked in healthcare before?" she asked. "No, I have a journalist background," I began. Maureen looked at me and began to roll her eyes as if she had given up hope.

"You will work with Maria in the morning to assist the patient with their washes," Maureen muttered before heading to the nurse's room to collect her drug trolley.

Maria stood in the female bay I was working in with her care trolley filled with pads, washcloths, and antibacterial soap. I walked into the bay and noticed that all the patients in the bay were sleeping. The first patient was Ethel, an eighty-nine-year-old lady. Deidre was over twenty stone and was admitted after a neighbor reported her to social services for not leaving her house in over a month. Deidre had become depressed following the death of her husband, and her body was covered in bedsores from staying in bed every day.

The second lady was Ethel, Ethel was admitted with confusion and general frailty, and her favorite pastime was singing songs from the '50s and 60's her favorite era. Ethel required one-to-one supervision dew to her recurrent falls.

The third patient was Julia, at 102 years old, she was the oldest lady I had interacted with and she was admitted due to an exacerbation in her diabetes condition. Julia was the most active elderly lady I had ever met and had a keen interest in helping others and was still remarkably very active in the ward.

The fourth patient was Sandra, Sandra was eight-five and was living with advanced dementia. Sandra required full hoisting in her chair and had lost the ability to communicate and would scream out to express her wishes. Sandra was admitted as her daughter was unable to physically look after her.

The fifth patient was Karen, a school dinner lady who had fully recovered from sepsis and was now awaiting discharge but was very frustrated in waiting for her medication and would often shout out and swear at colleagues.

The sixth patient was Mary, a sixty-seven-year-old lady admitted with palpitations and was later diagnosed with heart failure. As a team, we were asked to observe Mary closely when her family arrived as they were attempting to encourage her to sign her house over.

I then worked together with Maria to assist her with the patient washes. "Oh, look at him he only looks ten!" Deidre laughed. I felt nervous as we began to assist her with her wash. Deidre was covered in pressure sores, under her feet and on her elbows, and back that were at risk of turning necrotic. As we removed some of the dressing and washed Deidre with the warm water she yelled in pain.

"Oh, Tom don't stand there looking like a duck, place me the washcloths," she moaned. It felt hard to physically help Deidre move in the bed. The doctors believed her muscles had weakened from spending days in bed. "I don't like you, you always want to rush the wash," Deidre cried to maria. "I can't help you when I'm working with Tom, he has no idea about the routines here," Maria snapped.

It was then we assisted Sandra with her wash. Sandra was very distressed, and her dementia was so advanced, that she could not feed herself or pick up a drink and provided full care.

"Why don't you go and help out in the male bay, you're more suited there," Maria growled.

"I'm here to work with both male and female patients and this is the bay I am working in." I began. I immediately felt as soon as I worked with Maria that she did not want to work with a 'student' and had failed to support me, even though she had spent over twenty years on the ward as a care assistant.

We repositioned Sandra in the bed and helped to assist her with the wash. As we began to assist her, Sandra began to punch out at us and almost kicked me. As we helped Sandra, we had to hoist her into the rise and recliner chair. Maria became agitated at my lack of experience, "Right you are really getting on my nerves!" she scowled. Just then I was saved as my mentor Maureen reminded me that my student nurse meeting with other students in my cohort was in the library.

I felt like I had made a bad start, it was my first day working in a caring environment, and I felt unsupported by the staff. I sat in the student forum meeting with the placement manager Gill, who stood in her grey striped suit, holding a clipboard. Opposite to Gill were the two nursing students. Rebecca who had butterfly tattoos on her arms and neck and a lip ring and piercings on her nose, whilst the student nurse next to her Tracey, had curly red hair wrapped in a bun whilst her dark rimmed glasses covered her entire face.

"So how is it going, how is your morning going?" she asked.

"Not too bad, I have wicked as a healthcare assistant on the ward I'm on, so I already feel part of the team." Rebecca smiled; she then placed her legs on the table showing her black boots. I could see Gill's angry glare towards Rebecca, she had defied all the rules in the hospital dress code. "I have worked for twenty years as an auxiliary nurse, so this is a walk in the park for me. I worked here before you two were born!" Tracey whined.

"Well welcome to you all on your first placement, I want to thank you all for starting with us. I must remind you that nose piercings are not permitted, and tattoos are discouraged and should be covered up! If you need support please contact me, ask questions, and make the most of every opportunity," she smiled.

I felt so inexperienced in comparison to Rebecca and Tracey. Although Rebecca did not follow the dress code, she would later become a highly regarded heart specialist nurse. I felt I had so much work to do, I had so much to learn, and only three years to show my competency.

As I returned to the ward, I looked outside of the staffroom window and witnessed Maria smoking her cigar outside, she would often take regular breaks to speak to her friends in another ward. Debbie offered to show me around the ward, and we talked through paperwork, and she showed me how to empty catheters, and showed me the fire that existed on the ward. As I walked into my bay, I could see a stern-looking Maureen looking at her charts. "Oh, Tom please can you take the observations?" she asked.

I was nervous even taking the observations, every task was a brand-new experience. It took me over ten minutes to complete the observation for each patient. I was diligent in making sure I didn't make a mistake. There were so many challenges in the bay, Karen was desperate to go home, whilst Sandra and Ethel always required supervision.

"When am I going home, I want to get out of this awful place!" Karen stated. "I have contacted the pharmacist and your tablets will be ready by lunchtime, you will have to be patient," Maureen snapped.

I observed that Mary and Deidre were asleep, Maureen advised me that Ethel had kept them awake all night. I then walked over to Julia, who stood over her bed folding her clothes. I looked at the photos of Mary on her bed space, including a photo of her in her field with her two hundred school pupils as a headteacher. Whilst another photo showed Julia leading a dance glass to the over 80's in her community hall, another picture showed Julia getting ready for her beauty pageant shows in her late teens. I felt so fascinated talking to Julia learning all about her history, such as working in a factory during world war 2, her short time as a nun in her late twenties, and her later career as a cabaret singer. At 102 she was invincible, rushing around to attend to the needs of the other patients in the bay, including aiding Sandra's needs when she required support, such as assisting with her drinking.

Suddenly Ethel jumped up from her bed and burst out into song, "I can't help falling in love with you," she sang. I rushed over towards her as she appeared unsteady on her feet. Debbie rushed along to help me and placed her hand into Ethel's. "Where do you want to go my darling?" Debbie asked. "Toilet," Debbie replied. As Ethel reached the toilet, she hurried inside and slammed the door behind her, slamming the door in anger. We were very concerned as Ethel was unable to be left on her own, as she was very unstable on her feet. We tried to price the door open, but she refused to open the door. Then we heard the shower turn on and very quickly the water began to seep through the door, then we heard a loud thud on the floor, realizing that Ethel had fallen. Debbie quickly grabbed the hover bed machine from the equipment room. The hover bed was used to help patients who had a fall to reach safety.

We opened the door and Ethel was shaking on the floor, we had to gently roll her from side to side sliding the hover bed underneath it, as the machine turned on the bed and blew up into a mattress under one minute. Then we were able to move Ethel back into the bay, as she began to sing, 'Devil in disguise,' and she began to feel more settled.

"You will have to complete an incident room to document the fall." Maureen reminded me. It was then that Ethel led me into a waltz, I was nervous as she began to sing, 'hound dog' by Elvis. Ethel began to twirl in her nightdress as she believed she was wearing a ballgown. Ethel's behavior deteriorated very quickly over a sixth month period, and the staff believed she was unsafe to live on her own.

I watched from the bay as Maureen was deep in thought on the phone at the nurse's desk. I felt she was too busy to have a student. At every interval Maureen was busy, liaising with multidisciplinary staff, talking to relatives, and attending meetings with the ward manager. I felt almost childlike, I was nervous whenever I was left on my own, scared of making a mistake, scared of being judged by the staff.

I then watched as an agitated Karen appeared angry in her armchair, she was dressed in her blue suit with her suitcase packed. "Excuse me I have been waiting five hours for my tablets. How long will this take? Fucking hell!" Karen shouted. Karen was so frustrated after being on the ward for two months. I enquired from the busy pharmacist at the nurse's station, but she was too busy to speak to me.

It was then that I watched a concerned Maureen walking into the bay, as she noticed that Mary's family had arrived, and we had to carefully observe them, due to our suspicion that they were attempting to financially manipulate her. Maureen's son had drawn a curtain around her and was holding a pen in her hand to forge her signature on the deeds of the house. The ward manager told at the entrance of the curtain, "Please put the pen down, Mary clearly does not have the capacity," she warned. We finally had the evidence we needed to progress the safeguarding protocol to protect Mary, and her family quickly exited.

I felt so overwhelmed on my first day in the ward, I had watched so many health programs on television, and I felt like I was participating in one. All the other staff members were so busy, the physiotherapists were rushing around with mobility equipment, the doctors were completing their ward round, and the cleaners were attempting to clean among the sea of people. On my first day, I was so unsure of what my role was, and I felt overwhelmed by all the new information I was taking in. I did not realize at the time, but communicating with the patients was a great learning tool. The buzzer suddenly rang, it was Deidre, and she asked to go to the toilet in the bed, and to use the bedpan. Debbie assisted me and due to her sheer weight, Deidre managed to crush the bedpan. "Oh Deidre, you should really try mobilizing for the toilet.

"I'm far too depressed, the doctors believe that it's unsafe for me to go home, and I want to go home. If I go to a care home, all the decisions will be made for me," Deidre cried.

"We will help you, Deidre we are here to support you," Debbie reminded her. It was then that Deidre held onto my hand and thanked me for making time to talk to her. Talking to Deidre helped me to see the true essence of being a nurse, being there for students at their most vulnerable.

The visitors came in later in the afternoon for an allocated time slot which left me apprehensive. Suddenly the visitors were asking me a range of questions, "How has Sandra been?" Asked her concerned daughter. "Why has Karen been waiting for her discharge all day?" "Is Deidre going to be coming home?" asked the neighbor. I had to relay every question to Maureen.

At mealtime, we had to reposition the patients to make them comfortable and settled for feeding. I sat next to Sandra and assisted her with her small puree meal, I gazed at her food chart and observed that she only had a few spoonfuls of her meal, and she took just one spoonful of her roast meal. As soon as she received her chocolate smoothie pudding, she devoured every spoonful. I had watched how vulnerable able she was and how she was so dependent on me helping her with almost every task. For years I had worked in an office in a cold environment, but working in the hospital made me feel like I was part of a community trying to work together, to support patients to reach the best outcome.

After the meals were finished my mentor Maureen completed the drugs round, apologizing to me that she had been so busy during the shift covering for the staff shortage. Maureen was a single mother of five children, and worked as a nurse for four shifts a week. I felt through my placement that Maureen was tough on me at times, but she had found it very difficult being a mother of four children and working unsociable hours. Maureen had a lot of knowledge to share having worked as a nurse for ten years.

Going into university was a great way to speak to other students, to share our experiences, and learn the theory behind nursing. In my first placement which was six weeks, I spent half of my time between University and the hospital setting. In my cohort of nursing students, we had students from a range of backgrounds, including school leavers, people changing careers, and students who wanted to progress into senior roles in their healthcare career.

During the lectures, I found it humorous seeing the characters of the students come to life in the lectures. Simon, the sixty-year-old journalist looking for a change of career, would sit with his clipboard, and his red glasses brimmed on his nose. During the lectures he would seek to question the theories of the lectures, asking them where they got their evidence from and would often create heated arguments. Then there was Alice, a twenty-four-year-old ex-hairdresser who would often distract the tutors with her behavior. Alice would come to lectures dressed in multicolored dresses and would sit painting her nails and chewing bubblegum.

The lecturers would often ask her a question, and she would shoot back a look of deep confusion, and shouted, "I beg your pardon.

Then there was Mandy, a fifty-year-old single mother of two who would arrive late for every lecture, and Mandy would drive her black jeep into the university filled with rubbish. Mandy would sit at the back and would often consume a three-course meal. Sometimes I would turn around and see a cloud of smoke coming from her fresh turkey meal she heated up in the student kitchen. By the end of the lecture, Mandy could be found in a deep sleep snoring.

The best part of being at University was catching up on much-needed sleep. Most days on placement I would wake up at 5am, and arrive home at 7pm exhausted often falling asleep on the sofa. Every Friday my cohort of students would get together and grab an ice cream and go to the cinema. It was a great way to unwind and relax after a week of long lectures.

Chapter 6: District nursing

In the second year, I learned more about the social determinants of health and community nursing, and I was excited to work in my community placement with the district nursing team. The stark difference between working in the ward and working in the community was clearly apparent. The early mornings, long hours and unpredictable nature of work were replaced by 9-am-4pm starts, and a relaxed working environment, with more time to spend with patients.

I was nervous on my first day at the district nurse's office, as I arrived with my satchel with my notebook, pens, folder, and crackers and cheese. As I walked into the district nurse I was startled, surrounded in silence, watching the sea of nurses sitting at their desks, quietly organizing notes for the day.

In the corner was Abigail Miller, a young 24-year-old nurse, Abigail stood up in her blue sequined outfit.

"Hi Tom, I am Abigail and your mentor, you are my first student," she smiled.

"Nice to meet you," I began. I could tell within the first few minutes that Abigail was enthusiastic about being a mentor, she presented me with a nursing handbook, a booklet of common nursing terms, and the routine of the day.

"We are a virtual ward service, we support patients who have recently been discharged from hospital. Between 9 am and 10 am we prefer for our day and we may receive phone calls from the clients. Then between 10 am-4 pm we visit the patients before returning to the office at 4 pm to complete our notes," she began.

It was then that I saw the list of patients we would see during the day. The patients ranged from a lady due for a diabetes check to a lady requiring inclusion in a care home, to a welfare visit to a man who was admitted due to making several suicide attempts.

At 9:10 am the phone started to ring, and Abi passed me the headphones for the phone so I could listen to the phone call.

"Hello Abigail, how are you? She asked

"Good Jean, how are you?" Abigail asked.

"I need help with a crossword first letter is F second and third is U C-"

"Oh, Abbie will come and visit you tomorrow we can discuss your holiday," Abigail stated.

"Hold on what did you have for your breakfast?" she asked.

Abigail explained that Jean called every morning, even though she was now fit for discharge, she rang just for company.

It was then that we received a phone call from Dana, the first patient we were due to see for her diabetes check. Dana had recently been diagnosed with Alzheimer's disease and appeared confused at times on the phone.

"Good morning is that Abi?"

"Good morning Dana, yes, it is Abi, I am due to see you at 10 am today, how can I help you?" Abi asked.

"Oh, it's terrible my toilet! I tried to flush it but now there is a flood there's been a blockage, oh Abi please come it smells rotten."

"Dana I will be at your house straight away, please don't panic." Abi looked on in terror, and we quickly exited the office and entered her yellow sports car. We appeared to zoom across the motorway as we made our way to Dana's house. As Dana opened the boot, I saw her district nurse kit, filled with wipes, dressings, and PPE equipment. Dana quickly passed me gloves and an apron and a waste bag to wrap around our feet to enter Dana's house.

As we entered Dana's house she was visibly shaken and began to cry, "Thank you both for coming so soon your angels!" she smiled. As we went upstairs, we could see that she had flooded the bath and smeared the feces over the walls. I watched as Dana put several towers on the floor, and helped to clean the wall, before ringing the plumber to assess the situation further.

We walked downstairs and sat next to Dana as Abigail made her a cup of tea. We observed how Dana was struggling at home, the work surfaces were covered in mold, the food was out of date in the kitchen, and visibly Dana's clothes were ripped and dirty. Dana's daughter had been on vacation for over a month, and Dana showed how much she was struggling to care for herself.

"Dana, I think you could benefit from extra help in your home I understand your finding it difficult," Abigail began,

"I don't need a social worker, I mean you can fix toilets, you're a Jack of all trades," she smiled.

"We just need to make sure your safe at home, you may benefit from carers,"

"I'm not going into a care home as God is my witness, I want to stay at home!" Dana roared.

It was so sad to see how desperate Dana was to hold onto her independence, but her dementia condition would eventually leave her with the ability to lack mental capacity. Abigail took Dana's blood observations and blood sugars, and they were all within the normal range despite her unhealthy diet. As we left Abigail stated she would report her concerns to Dana's social worker to promote her safety.

We then sped off in the sports car continuing our journey through the day, I put the window down and enjoyed taking in the cool breeze. I thought about my peers working in the ward environment, completing their washes, and responding to the constant ringing of the buzzers. We arrived at the Arnold Grove nursing home at 10 am, it was a sixty bedded nursing home with over sixty residents. Abigail had several patients to see at the home to administer insulin. Abigail had organized for me to spend time in the dementia circle time, an activity group to support patients with dementia.

As we entered the home, we were greeted to a birthday party, Geoffrey who was living with dementia was celebrating his 100th birthday. He was dressed in a smart business suit, with a shiny red birthday hat, and he held onto an assortment of cards. Geoffrey was surrounded by pictures of his time as a doctor in London. Suddenly the care home staff walked in with a three-foot tiered birthday cake with sparklers attached, I felt I had gatecrashed a birthday party.

It was then that the care manager organized fifteen residents to attend the dementia activity group. Abigail left me alone in the group with the performer. "Right everyone, we are going to be singing some of our favorite songs. Today, first we will sing daisy. As the group started to sing the elderly lady Rose sitting next to me held onto my hand and clenched it tightly. "Look everyone, I have a new boyfriend," she yelled. I watched as the other residents cheered and laughed.

Suddenly the lively performer dressed as a school cheerleader introduced me to the group, "Right this is Tom everyone he has come to assist us in our activity group. Tom, would you like to sing for us? You can sing and we can follow." She began.

It was then that Rosie grabbed her guitar and sat at the stand, waiting for me to sing. I sat, nervously, on the chair and began to sing, "When the night has come." It was then that the elderly group sang, 'stand by me,' It was interesting to see the effect of music on the residents living with dementia. One man who was unable to speak was able to sing in and join in the music. It was then that Rosie walked around to each person in the circle, to take their hands and encourage arm movements to the 50's music. The last activity included a parachute activity in which each resident had to hold onto a side of the parachute and wave it slowly in the air. As the activity finished the elderly lady next to me kissed me on the face leaving a lipstick mark. It was then that Abigail arrived, and we departed on our journey for the rest of the day. As I sat in the car Abigail described her history in her nursing career. Abigail worked in a nursing home for two years and then spent five years as a critical care nurse before moving into the community sector.

The next house we arrived at was Audrey's house. Audrey was a sixty-year-old woman living with chronic COPD and end-stage heart failure. We entered Audrey's house and entered through the key safe. Audrey lived in a picturesque Edwardian cottage hidden by Oak trees. As we entered, I looked in shock at the dining room which was filled with so many animals and creatures. Audrey lay in her hospital bed in the corner of the room. In the room were two parrots in cages, six black cats, two rockrilers, and three rabbits. I always struggled around animals and felt instantly uncomfortable. Audrey had carers four times a day, and Abigail came to administer her insulin injection and end of life medication. As we walked over to Audrey, she watched the film Calamity Jane attached to the ceiling. "Oh, look you brought a man to see me, he is like a second-hand version of Elvis," she laughed. "I guess," Abigail smiled.
"How have you been," I asked.
"I have accepted my prognosis. I have a matter of months left but I am happy, the carers come to see me and hoist me into the chair, and I get to spend time with the animals. They are my only company, my only friends." Audrey smiled.

We observed Audrey scratching her leg, and as she uncovered her trousers, we noticed her legs were red raw and required a dressing. Abigail left the room to grab the dressings from the car.

I was petrified watching the animals around the living room, the rockrilers sat on the couch, stirring, their yellow eyes glared into mine. The parrots began to shout 'hello,' and the cats crawled around my legs. I could feel my heart pound and sweat poured down my face. As Abigail came back, I completed the non-touch technique to complete the dressing, nervously, knowing that Abigail was watching every nursing task I completed.

It was then that Audrey burst out into song singing the black hills of Dakota, and I watched as Abigail sang together, showing how she had a great rapport with her patients. Suddenly both the rockrilers started barking, in shock, I jumped back banging my head on the wall, Abigail and Audrey burst out laughing.

"Arr bless him he must be a virgin Abi, do you have a girlfriend?" Audrey asked. Instantly my face turned in embarrassment. You could always rely on patients to speak their minds at the most awkward moments. After the dressing was completed, we helped to reposition patients in the bed, to reduce the risk of pressure sores, then Abigail administered the end of life medication. I was so happy when we could finally leave the animal sanctuary.

The final house we visited was 90 years old Derek's house, who lived in a grand mansion on his own. Derek was admitted to the hospital a month previously after taking an overdose of paracetamol tablets. Our visit to Derek was based around providing him a list of local support groups, reviewing his medication, and providing emotional support. Part of the role of being a nurse was supporting the whole patient's physical and mental wellbeing.

As we walked inside Derek's mansion, we marveled at the grand dining room, which had a white grand piano and black leather seats and a ten-foot cinema screen in the corner. The dining room doors lead to the scenic ten-acre garden with a waterfall feature. Derek was a retired police sheriff and had worked as a policeman for over forty years. Although Derek had amassed a great fortune, he lived alone in his grand mansion. Twenty years previously Derek went for a drive in his jeep with his wife and daughter, and crashed into a tree causing his wife and daughter to die, as they were not wearing his seat belts.

Traumatized by what he had experienced, Derek cut family friends out of his life and became a recluse. After attempting suicide, he was sent to a psychiatric ward for assessment.

Derek explained that he had visited a counselor, and had undergone cognitive behavioral therapy which he felt supported him.

Abigail provided Derek with a range of support groups and had reviewed his medication.

"I sat here in my rocking chair for over twenty years, grieving, crying, remembering the positive times with my family. The suicide attempt was a way of escaping from my grief and trauma. In the hospital, I was treated with compassion by the nurses, for the first time I was being listened to. I was connected to a support group of people who had been through a similar experience, it saved me." Derek smiled as tears fell from his face. "At the virtual ward, we will continue to monitor you for over a year. If you require any help or advice call the district nurse office," Abigail smiled.

Visiting Derek opened my eyes to the experience that many patients in the hospital were going through, loneliness and isolation. Derek had spent so many years not interacting with another human being and was confined to the prison of his mansion. Abigail's involvement helped me realize the important work of nurses in being calm, patient, and attentive listeners to vulnerable patients.

Abigail was a very caring and knowledgeable nurse, I felt so supported and I learned so much about the community settings and how to care for vulnerable patients in their own setting.

After my community placement, my whole life was about to change forever.

On September 11th, 2001 my life was about to change forever.

I was revising for my anatomy and physiology exam and covered my bedroom in pictures of different parts of the anatomy.

As I walked down the creaky wooden stairs, I could hear the house phone ringing. It was my brother Ben talking in a muffled, anxious, and frightened tone.

"Mum, Mum, are you ok? Have you seen the news?"

"Ben, what's wrong? You sound panicked," Mum sighed as she sat on the couch. It was then that Mum turned on the television and on sky news the horror unfolded. We observed that a plane had crashed into the twin tower, the North tower, the building which Ben worked in. I collapsed to the floor, I was numb and in shock.

"Oh my God Ben, please tell me your outside!" Mum gasped.

"We are trapped inside, the firefighters are coming up Mum we're going to be ok, I just want to tell you and Dad and Tom, I love you all, please don't panic."

"No, Ben what are you doing now, you need to get out immediately!" mum panicked.

It's not safe to leave, the security team has said we need to stay here before the rescue team arrives. Listen, Mum, I have to go but I will call you back." he hung up.

I watched as my Mum threw the phone on the floor in shock and collapsed onto the sofa in a state of terror. In the background of Ben's phone call, I could hear the crying from his co-workers, the muffled cries for help, and the panicked phone call. I Felt Like I was watching a thriller, it looked so surreal, I wanted to believe it was a stunt, I wanted to wake up from this terrible nightmare. I believed that people could survive, I thought it was a terrible accident, the news reporters were confused, the scenes of people watching the towers in disbelief appeared on the screen. I observed Mum ringing Dad, her voice shaken and hands trembling.

I quickly ran to the kitchen to grab a glass of water before I sat on the couch in the living room. The room was filled with silence, then it happened the first tower fell, I felt my heart pounding against my chest, I was

sweating in fear.

The phone rang.

"Ben are you safe? Please tell me you're safe," Mum pleaded.

"A part of the roof has caved in, we are trapped here, but the firefighters

are coming up."

"What can you see? You're going to be ok," Mum warned.

"All I can see is a cloud of smoke, all we know is the North tower has

collapsed," Ben cried. In the background, I could hear the harrowing cries

from the co-workers and the screams for help.

"Mum is Tom there?"

"Yes," Mum gasped.

"Any money I have you both can have access to I have made an advance

will. I want to thank you and Dad for always supporting me. It was my

dream to work and study in America and you helped me achieve it. Tom, I

know we didn't always get on, but I am so proud of you, Mum tell Dad-"

It was then that the phone line cut, Mum desperately tried to ring Ben back,

but he did not answer. Ten minutes later we watched as the south tower collapsed. I burst into tears, knowing that Ben was trapped in the tower. I watched as Mum stared at the television screen vacantly.

After that we never heard from Ben again, he was presumed dead, but his body was never found.

For weeks and months, we examined photographs and videos of people jumping from the tower and video footage on various websites. Mum and Dad even traveled to New York to assist in the search rescue. It was the most devastating experience of my life. I became a recluse and decided to hide away in my bedroom in complete despair. I had taken a six-month break from my nursing course, and after family counseling and a month break in Cornwall, I was ready to face my final year.

The final year of my nursing year was met with many challenges, I had to become more emotionally resilient in the face of my brothers passing, and work full time, all whilst coping with the demands of the coursework. Since my brother's passing, I felt at times I wanted to give up on being a nurse, but I had to carry on.

Chapter 7: Final placement.

My final nursing placement was in a small Accident and Emergency, and a lot of pressure was put on me to achieve the skills I had learned during the three years. My mentor Annie, was forty-three and had spent over twenty years in the Emergency Department and was a student coordinator. Life in the Emergency department was so fast paced, often when I would go on my break and come back, patients would be moved to another ward or discharged. I was given cubicles 1 and 6 to look after, and a patient in the side room. All the doctors would congregate around the nurse's station and I would witness the nurses running around the ward.

On this day, it was early silent in the department. Only a few patients were on the ward, whilst Annie was at the desk managing the ward as Senior nurse on the shift. I was being observed from afar and with little supervision. I would run through the protocol of the tasks, I needed to complete including patient admissions, ECG readings, and clinical observations. I found accidents and emergencies particularly hard to work on as there was little opportunity to plan care, and I would have to use my initiative to respond to emergency situations.

Suddenly my first two patients arrived, John Sampson, an eighty-five-year-old consultant admitted following attempting suicide at his GP clinic and was found collapsed in the toilet, as he attempted to cut his wrists. John was sixty-five, and sat in his blue business soon, his curly grey hair covered his face. As soon as I assisted John onto the hospital trolley the second patient arrived, Jean Carter. Jean Cater was eighty-five, and was admitted after a fall in the kitchen, reporting that she felt dizzy.
I noticed the paramedics had placed dressings on John's wrist, he requested me to close the cubicle curtains.

"I just want to ask for some privacy please, I used to work here, and I do not want to cause a scene. I've just been having a tough time; I was the career for my mother who recently passed away. I should have sought help for my mental health, but the situation has escalated. After taking John's observations, I asked the care assistant Julie to observe John, whilst I called the mental health team to come to assess John.

I attended then to Jean, whilst being aware I could have more admissions at any second. Jean sat up in her hospital trolley wearing her pink dressing gown and black boots, whilst her son Derek sat next to her sobbing.

"I understand you had a fall in the kitchen, and you were feeling ill?" I asked.

"Well Mum has not been looking after herself she has been drinking two bottles of vodka a night and eating unhealthy foods despite being diabetic." He cried.

I then took Jean's blood sugar and noticed it was very high and took a blood test to send off for sampling.

"Listen, young man, I really shouldn't be here, I just want to go home."

"We just need to run a few tests, just to make sure you are ok, you may be admitted to the ward," I added.

I then rushed over to the ward doctor sitting by the Phone, so calm and composed in his pink suit. "Doctor Jean's blood sugar is 20 and her blood pressure is very high can you please assess her, Now!" I ordered, assertively, as he sheepishly put his phone in his pocket. It was then then that my patient in the bedroom pressed his Buzzer.

Tanzer was from Romania and spoke very little. It was confirmed that he had swine flu, so I had to wear the PPE equipment. I walked into Tamzer's room and looked on in shock. The room was filled with open crisp packets, pots of half-eaten yogurts, and a stack of toilet roll.

"Excuse me, man I need a toilet, get my stick, hurry up!" he shouted. I watched as Mr. Tanzer ordered me, I felt like a butler.

"Pick me up, help me to the toilet!

I explained I could not pick him up and watched as Tanzer lifted himself up to reach his Zimmer frame, "you bastard English no listen, pass me four toilet rolls," he ordered, as he reached the toilet he slammed the door in my face. We had our carer assistant call in sick, so I had to complete many tasks on my own. Outside I saw a few of Tanzer's family member's waiting outside.

"Only two visitors," I warned. I watched with apprehension as over ten family members entered the room, "Two I give you five!" yelled the elderly lady.

As I left the room I watched as the doctor was now assessing my patients and it was time for me to take my break. As I sat in the staff room, Annie came in to check if I was ok and to congratulate me on my hard work. I worried about the patients whilst I was on my break, I needed to keep busy to keep my mind off my brother, I did not like being left with my own thoughts.

After my break, I was surprised to see that already four more patients had arrived into my remaining cubicles, whilst Lizzie the agency nurse helped to admit them.

Rita was sat in a cubicle, knitting, admitted after being found wandering on the streets. Michael at twenty-six, was admitted after fracturing his knee following a late-night game of football. In cubicle six was Michael dressed in his nice outfit and was admitted with severe cuts to his hand after falling off his motorbike, In Cubicle seven was Christopher a seventy-six-year-old man, admitted due to collapsing in his home, and it was later discovered that he had suffered a left-sided stroke.

John had been assessed by the mental health team as unsafe to go home and was transferred to a psychiatric unit, whilst Jean was moved to the diabetic ward for further assessment.

I felt so under pressure to complete my tasks and felt my head spinning. I had to complete the care plan, admissions, and all the clinical assessments in a timely manner. I was still so hungry and thirsty but there was no time to meet my own needs.

I sat with Rita to complete a mini mental health assessment, which included asking her a series of questions to assess her mental state.

I gave Rita a copy of the assessment and asked her a raise of questions including naming animals, recalling information, and completing simple sums. Rita sat scribbling on the back of the assessment sheet. Rita showed that she was struggling with her short-term memory being unable to recall time, place and date. When I Picked up Rita's assessment sheet, I witnessed that she had written, 'she'll be coming around the mountains when she comes.' I realized that Rita required a further assessment and a possible admission to a general medical ward.

I then went to assess Michael, he began to scream out in pain, I took his observations and discovered that his temperature and blood pressure was very high. Doctor Clive came over and as he examined Michael, he expressed that he felt he needed major surgery and he was rushed to theatre for emergency treatment.

I then walked over to Mat. Mat was six foot seven and dressed in his leather outfit. He had long hair and wore large black oval sunglasses. I examined the glass in his hand and carefully began to remove it. "I don't really want a male nurse, I want a female nurse," he groaned.

"I can try"

"Just get on with it!" He groaned. As I removed the glass from Matthew's hand he began to scream out in pain and groaned in despair.

"What a nuisance, you took forever!" I watched as he angrily moved from the chair.

"Hold on you can't just go, you need further assessment," I warned.

Matthew did not listen, and he proceeded to self-discharge. It was so difficult as a student nurse to cope with angry behavior and so important to remain emotionally resilient.

I then went to assess Chris with the doctor. I could see that he had a facial droop. He looked petrified as he was unable to move his arms. I covered him in two extra blankets as he was shivering. The CT scan had confirmed that a stroke had occurred. I held onto Christopher's shaking hand, "You're going to be ok, I'm here for you," I whispered. I could see how petrified Christopher was as tears rolled down his cheek. Chris was admitted a year previously and had a triple heart bypass and lived alone following the passing of his wife. The doctor confirmed that Chris would be moving to the stroke assessment ward.

I sat next to Chris and explained where he would be going to. As I looked ahead, I could see the nurses rushing around, and I was filled with a vision of the twin towers. Suddenly, I could see the smoke and my brother saying his final goodbye. I looked at my fob watch with the words, 'keep going' engraved with my brother's initials, and I promised to never let him down.

I passed my final assessment and was now successfully registered as a general nurse. For over twenty years I have worked on a variety of different wards and I am now a lead nurse on an ophthalmology nurse. Before I started my nurse training, I was shy and apprehensive, after completing my nurse training, I became a stronger and more resilient person. I am now a student placement coordinator, and have enjoyed working with several students in helping them to complete their training.

Lucy's Nursing journey

Chapter 8: New Beginnings

In 2002 I began my nurse training and my life changed forever. A year before starting my nurse training, my life changed forever. I met my husband Sean at university at 19, and five years later we married in a luxurious ceremony in Florida. A year later we welcomed twins Daisy and Alice to our family. We lived happily for over five years, Sean worked as a lecturer and I worked as a secondary English teacher. At the age of 30, my life changed forever, and I felt like I would never recover from the situation. I woke up on a warm August afternoon and found a note on our bedside table explaining that he wanted to file for divorce and he was going away to live with his partner in Devon, after that morning I never saw him again. I was now a single Mum, recently made redundant, and realized I couldn't keep up the payments of the house and had to move in with my parents. I felt like my life was falling apart, everything I had worked hard for had been shattered.

Whilst I lived with my parents and felt hopeless, I realized I needed a change of career, a change in my life. I saw a poster on a billboard calling out for nurses and I applied. I wanted to make a difference and help others who were vulnerable.

I was so thankful that my parents were willing to help with childcare duties, to enable me to carry out my nurse training. I was so excited to commence my first placement on a stroke ward. The stroke ward was a busy thirty bedded ward, with an assessment center and a rehab gym. As I entered the ward I watched in awe at the speed of the nurses in each section. The assessment section and ward were kept separate, and I was to spend most of my time on the ward. The ward environment was thriving, and busy, the patients required one to one supervision and the nurses stayed in their bay for most of their shift.

My Mentor was Flo, a Forty-two-year-old nurse from the Philippines with over twenty years of experience. Flo was the most experienced nurse I knew, Flo had advanced medical nursing, and was an advanced clinical practitioner but preferred the ward environment. The ward had great morale, all the staff was supportive of students, and help was always on hand when you needed it.

On my first shift, I was working in a bay with five patients who were all admitted following a stroke. The first patient was Mena, a seventy-nine-year-old lady who was unable to regain any movement following the stroke and lost the ability to communicate.

In the second bed was Dawn, a fifty-two-year-old lady who collapsed during an assembly at school, and it was later discovered that she had a stroke. Dawn was very nervous and apprehensive, following the stroke, and struggled to come to terms with what happened.

In the third bed was Eilish, Eilish was admitted with left-sided weakness coinciding with her dementia. Since Eilish was admitted she had smashed windows with a walking stick, poured cold water over a patient, and threw an assortment of fruit at the junior doctors.

Tess was the youngest patient in the ward at the age of fifty she was a highly skilled artist. The pictures on her wall were completed with intricate detail with acrylic paints and charcoal. Tess was also a single mother with four children.

The majority of my first placement revolved learning basic care in nursing, and I assisted the healthcare assistant with Shirley with the washing and dressing tasks. The first patient I supported was Dawn the headteacher. "Hi, Dawn I'm Lucy I am looking after you today, is it ok if I can help you with a wash?" I asked. I watched as Dawn began to cry. It was then I realized I was put in such a responsible position Supporting this successful businesswoman who was in shock following the shock.

Dawn required full assistance with washing and dressing, and we had to hoist her into the chair. I was happy to help Dawn look presentable and I was able to brush her hair and apply her perfume. "Dawn we are here for you today if you require any more support please call us." I began. I assisted Shirley in helping Dawn reposition in her chair with the pillows. I was nervous but remained calm and composed at all times.

It was then that we walked up to Eilish, as she sat in her chair, I watched as she stared vacantly into the distance in her pink dressing gown. "Hi Eilish can I help you with the wash?" I asked. Suddenly Eilish poured the water over my face," buzz off you fat cow!" She yelled.
It was then that Shirley rushed to my assistance, "ok Eilish we will come back in an hour to help you with a shower," Shirley added.

It was then that we walked over to help Mena with her wash. Mena had photos of her thirty Grandchildren. Mena's bedside was filled with positive pictures of attending graduations, attending birthday parties, and playing with her Grandchildren on the beach. As we assisted Mena I watched as she was able to point to pictures such as a brush, toothbrush, and toilet in her visual communication book. As we hoisted Mean in the chair she smiled and kissed our hand. It was so difficult having a one-way conversation.

A half an hour later I assisted Eilish into the showroom for her wash. I was filled with apprehension, as I had never interacted with a person with dementia. I was unsure of the correct communication methods. I watched as Eilish sat nervously on the chair. I turned the shower on and suddenly Eilish erupted into anger and pushed me against the wall hitting me on the head.

"You silly bitch, you fat cow, you stole my money, give it back now!" she roared. Meanwhile, the shower head was rolling on the floor and the water caused a river to form out from under the door. Suddenly Flo and Shirley arrived and were able to instantly diffuse the situation. Flow gently took Eilish by the hand and was able to coax her to her armchair by tempting her with a cup of tea.

I was amazed by Flo's care and consideration, Flo assisted me with completing the care plans, explained the conditions of patients in greater detail, and encouraged me to participate in the ward round.

As Elish's behavior on the ward worsened I was asked to stay in the bay at all times as a safety precaution.

I watched as Tess sat in her Simpsons pajamas. Tess was able to point to letters to ask me a question, she asked me if I had children and my age. I admired the pictures her children had drawn, with the words, 'I love mummy' scrawled on the page. It was then that I worked with the occupational therapist by helping her to hold a pencil in her hand and to start drawing. I could see how hard she was trying to keep the pencil on the page, as the stroke had disrupted her cognitive ability to draw.

Then the postman arrived with a package for Dawn, the package contained a plant and a card from all the teachers in her skill sending their wishes. I watched as Dawn's face lit up in happiness. Having a stroke has such a strong psychological impact on patients.

I watched as Dawn helped me to prioritize the patient's care including making sure patients were repositioned every two hours, making sure care plans were completed, and ensuring that the personal needs of patients were met.

I fell on my first day like I was in a fishbowl, the stroke ward was such a busy environment with the sounds of buzzers ringing constantly, and the constant shouts of patients asking for help.

Just before the end of my shift as I went to collect my coat from the handover room. The emergency buzzer in my bay began to ring. Claudia pressed the buzzer in my bay as she noticed that Tess was unresponsive. I watched as a sea of healthcare professionals ran with the crash trolley towards the bay. It was confirmed that Tess had gone into a cardiac rest. I watched as Flo led the CPR compressions, she was a natural leader, instructing other professionals and preparing the emergency equipment. After ten minutes the staff pronounced Tess dead. A tear rolled down my cheek, knowing that she was making good progress and knowing that her young children would not see her again.

As I arrived home that night my children were fast asleep in bed. It was the first time I had ever spent a whole day away from them. Although the hours of nursing were long, I made sure I cherished my time with my children. My first placement was a unique learning experience, I learned about basic nursing care, how to support patients who had just been diagnosed with a stroke, and how to record care. Flo imparted her knowledge onto me and helped to achieve a good grade.

Chapter 9: The dementia Clinic

In my second year of nursing, I was preparing for my community placement
and like every other nursing experience, I was apprehensive in entering
into a new setting. I was placed in a small dementia clinic attached to the

local hospital. My mentor Mazota revealed to me that she was 'forced' to have me as a student, and I felt very unwelcome in the setting from the start and regretted not speaking up about my concerns.

 The dementia clinic was a fast-paced setting, and over fifty patients would enter each day to be assessed for dementia or attended follow up treatments for their dementia. As a student, I would assist patients in taking the mini-mental health test and take their observations. With every consultation, I was able to observe the doctor's consultation.

I remember my first day and I observed Masota, stomping her feet, knowing that she had a student nurse. The sister of the clinic, Linda, welcomed me and directed me to the setting.

The first Patient to enter the clinic was Aldora, Aldora was eighty years old and an ex-army nurse. Aldora scored well on the memory test but the CT scan confirmed that she had frontotemporal dementia. I watched as Aldora sat in the clinical room with her husband, angry and frustrated.

Aldora's confusion made her believe that her husband was having an affair with her neighbor next door and she was unable to speak coherently. I watched as the doctor prescribed medication and support groups to Aldora's husband. During the consultation, Aldora stormed out with her satchel, angry that the doctor had 'misdiagnosed' her with dementia. The consultation with Aldora displayed to me how important it was for patients to get an early diagnosis. Aldora had refused to go to a doctor in over two years, and her condition deteriorated at that time.

I had fought so hard on my first day to impress Masota but I almost felt like the invisible student, and I was given no guidance.

The next patient was Mark, a 50-year-old man who attended the appointment with his daughter Sophie. Sophie was anxious as Mark presented with confusion for a year and it took so long to accept that there was a problem. I attempted to take Mark's observations but realized he was in a manic state, as Masota presented the mini-mental health test to him, Sophie guided me outside.

"I can't cope with looking after him anymore ever since his split from Mum his behavior has worsened, he is driving erratically drinking all the time and he is aggressive. We have had to call the police several times, as he often flies into a fit of rage and breaks items in the house. I can't cope anymore!" Sophie screamed. It was then that I guided Sophie to the visitor's room, and made her hot chocolate. It was so difficult to see people in such a distress stare, and it was even harder to offer families hope with an incurable condition.

As I walked into the GP consultation room, I witnessed how distressed Mark was as his dementia diagnosis was revealed, I watched as he stormed out of the room.

That afternoon I had a meeting with my mentor Masota in which I was tested randomly on my medical knowledge. I felt like she was trying to catch me out, trying to make me fail.

The next patient was a sixty-year-old lady called Lisa. Lisa attended the appointment with her neighbor Doris. Lisa was a renowned fitness instructor and nutritionist who had been struggling with her memory and was awaiting diagnosis. I witnessed how Positive Lisa was. As Lisa sat in the consultation room, the consultant stated that she had Alzheimer's disease. Lisa broke down in tears knowing that there was no cure and that she would one day be unable to continue her fitness classes. Although the consultant had prescribed Lisa with medications to slow down the progression, she was fearful of the progression of the condition. It felt empowering as a student nurse to offer her support groups and admiral nurse support.

My first day was challenging at the dementia clinic, and as time passed, I managed to change mentors which greatly improved my experience. On the first day of my placement, I shared a friendly conversation with a junior doctor called Jason. At the end of my placement, Jason presented me with a bouquet of flowers and invited me on a date to the harbor restaurant. I thought I would never find romance again when my husband walked out on me, and for the first time since he left me, I didn't feel so alone.

Chapter 10: The theatre Nurse

My final placement was the most difficult placement I was to encounter, but my mentor Andrew from Los Angeles was so supportive I knew I could get through it. I was placed in a theatre in a private hospital. My role included admitting patients, taking patients into theatre, supporting them in recovery, and finally on the ward.

I realized once I was in the theatre that I was more suited to working in a busy warm environment in the ward. I constantly felt cold in the theatre and would feel myself shivering as I walked out of the department.

The first patient I supported was Samantha, a sixty-year-old lady who was booked in for a total knee replacement. As soon as she came into the recovery room, I had to remove the tracheal tube and I watched as she slowly cried out in pain. I took Samantha's observations and her heart rate and blood were in the normal ranges. "Oh, help me please I can't beat this pain!" she cried. I watched as Anthony administered the morphine and I helped to move her to the ward.

I spent the remainder of my time in the ward overseeing the care of three postoperative patients. As I was on my management placement, I had to make sure the patients' observations were taken every fifteen minutes, that their care plans were updated and that their urine output was monitored.

The other patients I was supporting included Rachel, a sixty-five-year-old lady recovering from surgery. Rachel was very demanding and would press the buzzer constantly for support and would demand food and for her furniture to be rearranged.

The next patient was Eden, a 90-year-old lady admitted after a total hip replacement. Eden became very confused following her operation and the medical staff believed she was suffering from delirium. Eden would wander at night, take baths at 3 am, and sing at the top of her voice at 6 am. I was thankful Eden was in the room by the nurse's station, so that I could keep a close eye on her.

I was working on the shift with Jenny, a senior nurse who had worked in the private hospital for over thirty years. Jenny would constantly be off the ward smoking, you could see the steam of smoke evaporating from her hair. Every time I would ask Jenny for help, she would disappear or say that she needed to go to the bathroom.

I walked into Samantha's bedroom. The rooms in the private hospital were far more luxurious than the rooms on the NHS wards. The patients would sleep on double beds, the food was served on a silver tray, and there were fresh sheets and towels provided throughout the day.

I took Samantha's observations, and had witnessed that the morphine helped to control her pain. It was then that I looked at her face, it was green and that is when disaster struck. Suddenly Samantha vomited all over her sheets after finding a sandwich in her bag despite being told not to eat after surgery. I managed to help Samantha remain comfortabl,e and change into her nightdress.

"Oh, Louise I need your help, if my husband rings or arrives at the hospital I want you to refuse him entry to see me."
"Why?" I asked
"Well He paid for the surgery, but that is all I want, after I leave here, I am starting a new life In Devon, I cannot spend another day with him," she whined.
It was hard at times to follow the requests of patients, but we were always there to help in their darkest moments. That afternoon I spoke to Samantha's husband and he was very aggressive on the phone and in shock at her admission.

I walked into Rachel's room, and suddenly I was met with hundreds of her demands. "Oh Louise, can you move the television two meters to the light? The light from it is causing me a headache. Also, please can you bring me two glasses of water and a tray of biscuits," she yelled.

I often felt like a hotel attendant on the ward being expected to respond to every need of the patient.

As I walked into Eden's room I watched as she sat at her desk painting a poster with her assortment of paints. I stood in shock in the room and realized she had covered the floor and ceiling in paints, and she had managed to rearrange all the furniture in the room. I had received Eden's urine test results which confirmed she had a UTI.

An hour before the end of the shift a healthcare assistant discovered that Eden had taken a fall in the bath and was unresponsive, so she raised the emergency buzzer. I entered the room, along with Shirley, my mentor Anthony and Consultant Dr. Derek. Eden was laying on her back, I checked her airway and tried to rouse her, but she was unresponsive to voice and touch, and I could not feel a pulse. My mentor brought in the crash trolley, I felt a surge of adrenaline and started to do CPR, thirty compressions followed by a breath. My arms ached and sweat poured down my face.

At that moment I was so focused on my actions, the depth of my compressions, and the speed. I was given so much direction from the consultant Derek, after five minutes the other healthcare professionals took over. Den survived and regained consciousness that afternoon. I felt I had accomplished so much, and I showed that as a management student I was able to face direction.

Five years after my placement I now work as a senior nurse in a cardiology department. My relationship with Jason progressed and within a year after my training, we were married. My life as a Nurse has given me the independence I have longed for, and has given me a sense of purpose I have searched for.

My training as a student nurse changed my life forever. I started my nursing journey as a shy and quiet historian, and finished as an emotionally resilient person, equipped with the skills to change people's lives. Throughout my training years, I cared for my twin brother until he lost his battle with cancer as I commenced my final placement. Throughout my training, I gained the confidence to take the lead in CPR and emergencies, care for the critically ill, and support patients with a range of conditions. My most memorable placement as a student nurse was in the community setting. I worked with an eccentric Nurse called June who would dance with patients, sing with them, and build a strong rapport with them. June's vibrant personality and expertise inspired me in my nursing care and made the nurse I am today.

Chapter 11: Student Nurse Tips

Before you start a placement, it may be worth contacting the ward or department to check their routine and what is expected of you.

On each placement always identify to your mentor your learning needs and any skills you hope to gain.

Try to complete as many handovers as you can to help increase your confidence.

Try to work with other nurses on the ward, each nurse has their own set of skills and experience and you can gain so much.

If you have any concerns about your placement try to dissolve these with the ward manager. If your concerns arise raise this with your placement manager.

Make time to go to the student forum whilst on placement, it is a great time to meet other students and reflect on your experience.

.

If you experience a cardiac arrest on your ward, try to get involved even observing can help you.

Try to keep a diary after each shift it is important to reflect on your experience and it can be used as evidence.

Halfway through your placement, identify to your mentor any skills you need to gain. If you are put on an action plan find out the specific steps you need to take to pass.

To prepare for your placement read up on the area, this will help you in terms of understanding the conditions of patients.

If your placement setting asks you to provide feedback take this on board, positive or negative feedback can improve the experiences for future students.

At the end of each shift try to complete an activity or do something you enjoy for over an hour. In doing this you will be able to unwind.

If you have an assessment to complete during placement try to create a timetable of how you can fit in the extra study.

At university, always ask your personal tutor for advice, they are there to offer you advice.

If you fail an assignment, make sure you attend a tutorial and know the clear steps on how you can improve to achieve a pass.

If your university has a clinical skills room, make use of this as it is a great learning opportunity.

It may be helpful to revise with other students in the library sharing your knowledge with other students can be very helpful. Making your revision notes visual and vibrant can help you remember facts clearly.

The end

I hope you enjoyed the book, if you liked it please leave a review! Any

questions or advice please email me at buttinchris@aol.com

Printed in Great Britain
by Amazon